Spanish Diabetes
Phrasebook

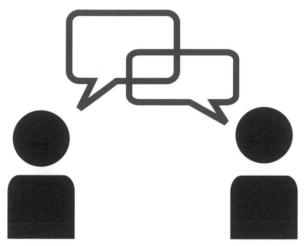

A RESOURCE FOR
Health Care Providers

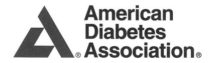
American Diabetes Association

Writer, Andrea Zaldivar; *Director, Book Publishing,* Robert Anthony; *Managing Editor, Book Publishing,* Abe Ogden; *Acquisitions Editor,* Victor Van Beuren; *Production Manager,* Melissa Sprott; *Translator,* Salud, Inc.; *Composition,* Jeff B. Johnston; *Cover Design,* Jeff B. Johnston; *Printer,* United Graphics, Inc.

Printed in the United States of America
1 3 5 7 9 10 8 6 4 2

The suggestions and information contained in this publication are generally consistent with the Clinical Practice Recommendations and other policies of the American Diabetes Association, but they do not represent the policy or position of the Association or any of its boards or committees. Reasonable steps have been taken to ensure the accuracy of the information presented. However, the American Diabetes Association cannot ensure the safety or efficacy of any product or service described in this publication. Individuals are advised to consult a physician or other appropriate health care professional before undertaking any diet or exercise program or taking any medication referred to in this publication. Professionals must use and apply their own professional judgment, experience, and training and should not rely solely on the information contained in this publication before prescribing any diet, exercise, or medication. The American Diabetes Association—its officers, directors, employees, volunteers, and members—assumes no responsibility or liability for personal or other injury, loss, or damage that may result from the suggestions or information in this publication.

♾ The paper in this publication meets the requirements of the ANSI Standard Z39.48-1992 (permanence of paper).

ADA titles may be purchased for business or promotional use or for special sales. To purchase more than 50 copies of this book at a discount, or for custom editions of this book with your logo, contact the American Diabetes Association at the address below, at booksales@diabetes.org, or by calling 703-299-2046.

American Diabetes Association
1701 North Beauregard Street
Alexandria, Virginia 22311

DOI: 10.2337/9781580403337

Library of Congress Cataloging-in-Publication Data

Spanish diabetes phrasebook : a resource for health care providers / American Diabetes Association.
    p. ; cm.
  Includes index.
  ISBN 978-1-58040-333-7 (alk. paper)
  1. Diabetes--Terminology. 2. Spanish language--Conversation and phrase books (for medical personnel) I. American Diabetes Association.
  [DNLM: 1. Diabetes Mellitus--Phrases--English. 2. Diabetes Mellitus--Phrases--Spanish. 3. Diabetes Mellitus--Terminology--English. 4. Diabetes Mellitus--Terminology--Spanish. WK 15 S786 2010]
  RC660.S665 2010
  616.4'620014--dc22

                                      2009039851

CONTENTS

Introduction: Using This Phrasebook

This phrasebook was designed for physicians, clinicians, nurses, and other health care professionals working in emergency, urgent care, or other clinical situations where a Spanish translator is either hard to find or not available but the need for care is critical. It is not meant to replace a translator when treating a Spanish-speaking patient with diabetes. However, it does aim to provide translations for many of the questions that comprise a thorough examination of a patient with diabetes.

Question Construction

Most of the questions in this phrasebook are constructed to elicit either yes/no or simple, single-word answers, so that even users with little familiarity with Spanish can easily understand the responses. In those instances when a yes/no or one-word answer was not possible, multiple-choice options have been provided.

Use a Pen and Paper

When working with a Spanish-speaking patient, it is very helpful to have paper and a writing utensil available. This allows the patient to provide answers to questions in writing, which can make numbers and certain terms easier to understand. Writing instructions, terms, or numbers can also make it easier for the patient to understand you. For many, a second language is easier to read than it is to hear, so make sure you have the option to communicate in writing.

Alternate Terms or Phrasing

Because Spanish includes many regional dialects and variations, many terms have various translations. Many (though not all) of these variations are included here, presented in brackets [ ] with the original or more popular term underlined. At times, entire phrasings can vary based on dialect. In these instances, the alternate phrasing is presented in brackets.

Gender Variations

The spelling and pronunciation of many Spanish terms can vary based on the context of the sentence and the gender of the word it may modify. In instances where a word may have a different pronunciation or spelling based on gender variations, the alternate gender spelling is provided in parentheses

Greeting and Introduction

1. Good morning.
   Buenos días.

2. Good afternoon.
   Buenas tardes.

3. Good evening.
   [For early evening]
   Buenas tardes.

   [For late evening]
   Buenas noches.

4. Pleasure to meet you.
   Mucho gusto.

5. Pleasure to see you again.
   Es un placer volverle a ver.

6. My name is….
   Me llamo….

7. I will be your:
   Seré su…

        a. … doctor.
           …médico [doctor].

        b. … nurse.
           …enfermera.

c. ... nutritionist.

...nutricionista [especialista en nutrición, nutrióloga (-o)].

d. ... exercise physiologist.

...fisiólogo (-a) de ejercicios.

e. ... physician assistant.

...asociado [auxiliar, asistente] médico.

f. ... nurse practitioner.

enfermera (-o) de práctica avanzada [enfermera (-o) universitaria].

g. ... dietitian.

...dietista.

h. ... diabetes educator.

...educador en diabetes.

8. I will be working with you to help you with your diabetes.

Me ocuparé de ayudarle en el cuidado de la diabetes. [Le ayudaré y nos ocuparemos juntos del cuidado de su diabetes.]

9. May I ask you some questions about how you are feeling?

¿Me permite hacerle preguntas acerca de cómo se siente?

10. May I ask you some questions about your diabetes?

¿Me permite hacerle preguntas acerca de su diabetes?

Spanish Diabetes Phrasebook

Identifying the Patient

11. What is your name?

    ¿Cómo se llama?

12. What would you like me to call you?

    ¿Qué nombre prefiere?

13. What is your date of birth?

    ¿En qué fecha nació?

14. Have you been here before?

    ¿Ha estado aquí antes?

15. Who is your regular doctor?

    ¿Quién es su médico?
    [Quién es el médico que le atiende]

16. Do you know your medical record number?

    ¿Sabe el número de su historial médico?

    > a. [If yes] What is it?
    > ¿Cuál es?

17. Do you have insurance?

    ¿Tiene seguro?

    > a. [If yes] May I make a copy of
    > your insurance card?
    > ¿Me permite hacerle copia a su
    > tarjeta de seguro?

Medications and Allergies

18. What medications (and doses) do you presently take for diabetes?

    ¿Qué medicamentos (y dosis) toma actualmente para su diabetes?

19. Are any of these diabetes medications newly prescribed?

    ¿Le han recetado algunos de esos medicamentos recientemente?

    a. [If yes] Which ones are new to you?

       ¿Cuáles son los nuevos que toma?

20. Have any of the dosages or strengths of your diabetes medications been changed?

    ¿Le han modificado la dosis o la potencia [concentración] de los medicamentos que toma para la diabetes?

    a. [If yes] Which ones have been increased?

       ¿A cuáles se la han aumentado?

    b. [If yes] Which ones have been decreased?

       ¿A cuáles se la han disminuido?

    c. Were they decreased because:

       ¿Se las disminuyeron porque...

    i. they interfered with your kidneys?

    …le afectaban los riñones?

    ii. you became shaky or sweaty?

    …le daban temblores o sudaba?

    iii. you are pregnant?

    …estaba embarazada?

21. Do you take insulin?

¿Toma insulina?

    a. [If yes] How long have you been taking insulin?

    ¿Hace cuánto tiempo toma insulina?

    b. [If yes] What type of insulin do you take?

    ¿Qué tipo de insulina toma?

    [Refer to List of Diabetes Medications for possible Spanish drug name variants]

    c. [If yes] How much do you take and when?

    ¿Qué cantidad toma y cuándo?

22. What other medications do you take? How much do you take and when?

¿Qué otros medicamentos toma? ¿Qué cantidad toma y cuándo?

[Refer to List of Diabetes Medications
for possible Spanish drug name variants]

23. Are you taking medications from another
country without a prescription?

¿Toma medicamentos de otro país obtenidos
sin receta médica?

24. Do you take any herbs or dietary supplements?

¿Toma hierbas o suplementos [complementos]
dietéticos?

25. Do you have any allergies to food or medicine?

¿Hay alimentos o medicamentos que le
den alergia?

   a. [If yes] What food or medicine are
      you allergic to?

      ¿Qué alimentos o medicamentos
      le dan alergia?

26. Have you experienced any side effects from
your diabetes medications?

¿Ha tenido reacciones adversas a los
medicamentos que toma para la diabetes?
[¿Le han provocado efectos secundarios los
medicamentos que toma para la diabetes?]

   a. [If yes] Have you experienced.
      ¿En algún momento…

      i. Sweating?
        …ha sudado?

ii. Shakiness?
   …ha temblado?

iii. Diarrhea?
   …ha tenido diarrea?

iv. Vomiting?
   …ha vomitado?

27. Do any of your diabetes medications make you feel sick?

¡Toma medicamentos que le hagan sentirse mal?

28. What concerns you most about your diabetes right now?

    ¿Qué es lo que más le preocupa acerca de la diabetes ahora mismo?

   a. What to eat?

      ¿Qué comer?

   b. Eyes?

      ¿Los ojos?

   c. Feet?

      ¿Los pies?

   d. Heart?

      ¿El corazón?

   e. Kidneys?

      ¿Los riñones?

   f. High blood pressure?

      ¿La presión [tensión] alta? [¿La hipertensión arterial?]

   g. Slow-healing sores?

      ¿Llagas que toman tiempo en sanar [curarse]?

29. Does anything hurt right now?

    ¿Le duele algo ahora mismo?

30. Do you feel sick?

    ¿Se siente enfermo?

History of Present Illness (HPI)

31. How do you feel your blood glucose levels are doing?

    ¿Cómo cree que están sus niveles de glucosa [azúcar] en la sangre?

32. Do your blood glucose levels go up and down?

    ¿Le suben y bajan los niveles de glucosa en la sangre?

    a. [If yes] Do you know why?
       ¿Sabe por qué?

33. How long has your blood glucose been out of control?

    ¿Hace cuánto tiempo ha estado fuera de control su glucosa en la sangre?

    a. For one (1) month?
       ¿Uno (1) mes?

    b. For six (6) months?
       ¿Seis (6) meses?

    c. For one (1) year?
       ¿Un (1) año?

    d. For more than one (1) year?
       ¿Más de un (1) año?

34. Have you experienced "low sugars,"
or hypoglycemia?

¿Ha tenido "bajón de azúcar [niveles bajos de
azúcar]", o hipoglucemia?

35. Have you ever been sweaty or felt shaky?

¿Ha sudado o le han dado temblores?

    a. [If yes] Do you test your blood
       glucose when you feel this way?

       ¿Se hace la prueba de glucosa en la
       sangre cuando se siente de
       ese modo?

    b. [If yes] What blood glucose
       numbers do you see?

       ¿Qué números le salen para la
       glucosa en la sangre?

36. Would you like to learn about diabetes control
and good nutrition?

¿Quisiera saber más acerca del control de la
diabetes y de la buena alimentación?

37. Do you need to learn how to inject insulin?

¿Necesita aprender el modo de inyectarse
la insulina?

38. May I watch you inject insulin?

¿Me permite ver cómo se inyecta la insulina?

39. Where are you injecting? Please touch the parts of your body.

> ¿Dónde se la inyecta? Indíqueme la parte del cuerpo con la mano.

40. Do you take the next shot in a different location?

> ¿Se da la próxima inyección en otro sitio?

> a. [If yes] How do you move the shots around?
>
> > ¿Cómo hace para cambiar el sitio donde se inyecta?

41. Do you have a blood glucose meter?

> ¿Tiene un medidor de glucosa en la sangre?

42. Are you having any problems operating your blood glucose meter?

> ¿Tiene problemas al operar el medidor de glucosa en la sangre?

43. How old is your blood glucose meter?

> ¿Cuán viejo es su medidor de glucosa en la sangre?

44. How often are you checking your blood sugar?

> ¿Cuán a menudo verifica su nivel de glucosa en la sangre?

> a. Every day?
> > ¿Todos los días?

[If so] How many times a day?
   ¿Cuántas veces al día?

b. Every week?
   ¿Todas las semanas?

[If so] How many times a week?
   ¿Cuántas veces a la semana?

c. Rarely?
   ¿Rara vez?

[If so] How many times a month?
   ¿Cuántas veces al mes?

45. Can you buy strips and lancets?

   ¿Puede comprar las tiras y lancetas?

46. Is poor vision making it difficult for you to take care of your diabetes properly?

   ¿Se le hace difícil cuidarse bien la diabetes debido a problemas con la vista?

47. When did you last go to the eye doctor?

   ¿Cuándo fue la última vez que fue al oculista u oftalmólogo [especialista de los ojos]?

48. Has diabetes affected your ability to go to work?

   ¿Le ha afectado la diabetes en cuanto a su capacidad para trabajar?

49. How long have you had diabetes?

   ¿Hace cuánto tiempo tiene diabetes?

    a. One year?
       ¿Un año?

    b. More than one year?
       ¿Más de un año?

    c. More than five years?
       ¿Más de cinco años?

    d. More than ten years?
       ¿Más de diez años?

    e. More than fifteen years?
       ¿Más de quince años?

50. Is there diabetes in your family?

    ¿Padecen de diabetes en su familia?

51. Do you have high blood pressure?

    ¿Tiene presión alta [hipertensión arterial]?

52. What was your blood pressure the last time it was taken?

    ¿Qué presión sanguínea [tensión arterial] tuvo la última vez que se la tomaron?

53. Do you have high cholesterol?

    ¿Tiene colesterol alto?

54. Do you have a copy of your lab results?

    ¿Tiene copia de los resultados de laboratorio?

55. Do you use tobacco?

    ¿Usa tabaco?

[If yes]:

    a. Do you smoke cigarettes now?
    ¿Fuma cigarrillos ahora?

    b. Did you ever smoke?
    ¿Fumó alguna vez?

    c. How many cigarettes a day do you smoke?
    ¿Cuántos cigarrillos fuma al día?

    d. How many years have you been smoking?
    ¿Hace cuántos años fuma?

    e. When did you quit smoking?
    ¿Cuándo dejó de fumar?

56. Do you use recreational drugs?

¿Utiliza drogas recreativas [de uso social]?

    a. [If yes] Which drugs?
    ¿Qué drogas?

57. Do you know what an A1C is?

¿Sabe qué es un A1C [también llamada hemoglobina glucosilada o hemoglobina HbA1c]?

58. Do you know what your A1C level is?

¿Conoce su nivel de A1C?

59. Do you know what A1C level indicates that you are in "good" diabetes control?

¿Sabe qué nivel de A1C le indica que tiene un "buen" control de la diabetes?

60. When was your latest A1C check?

¿Cuándo verificó su A1C por última vez?

61. Do you know what your eAG is?

¿Sabe cuál es el promedio estimado de glucosa [glucemia media estimada] que usted tiene?

62. Do you exercise?

¿Hace ejercicios?

63. Do you walk, play soccer, swim, jog…

¿Camina, juega fútbol [balompié], nada, corre…?

64. Do you exercise every day?

¿Hace ejercicios todos los días?

65. Have you changed the way you eat?

¿Ha modificado la forma de alimentarse?

66. Do you count carbohydrates in the food you eat?

¿Cuenta los carbohidratos [hidratos de carbono] que se encuentran en los alimentos que come?

67. Have you ever been hospitalized?

    ¿Ha estado hospitalizado (-a) alguna vez?

68. Have you ever been hospitalized for your diabetes?

    ¿Ha estado alguna vez hospitalizado (-a) debido a la diabetes?

69. Why were you hospitalized for your diabetes?

    ¿Debido a qué de la diabetes estuvo hospitalizado (-a)? Was it because of: ¿Fue debido a…

    a. Low blood glucose?
       …bajos niveles de glucosa en la sangre?

    b. High blood glucose?
       …altos niveles de glucosa en la sangre?

    c. Your heart?
       …su corazón?

    d. Your feet?
       …sus pies?

    e. Other?
       …otros motivos?

70. Do you have heart disease?

¿Padece de enfermedades del corazón?

71. Have you ever had a heart attack?

¿Le ha dado un ataque al corazón [ataque cardíaco/infarto cardíaco /fallo cardíaco] alguna vez?

    a. [If yes] When did you have a heart attack?

      ¿Cuándo le dio un ataque al corazón?

72. Have you ever had heart surgery?

¿Le han hecho cirugía cardíaca alguna vez? [¿Le han operado alguna vez del corazón?]

    a. [If yes] When did you have heart surgery?

      ¿Cuándo le hicieron la cirugía cardíaca? [¿Cuándo le operaron del corazón?]

73. Do you have kidney disease?

¿Padece de enfermedades del riñón?

74. Do you need kidney dialysis?

¿Necesita hacerse diálisis renal [del riñón]?

75. Have you been told you will need a kidney transplant?

¿Le han alguna vez dicho que necesita un trasplante de riñón [trasplante renal]?

76. Are you on a special diet for your kidneys?

¿Sigue una dieta [un régimen] especial debido a sus riñones?

> a. [If yes] Has a doctor told you to avoid:
>
> ¿Un médico le ha pedido que evite…
>
>> i. Salt?
>>
>> …la sal?
>>
>> ii. Protein?
>>
>> …las proteínas?
>>
>> iii. Potassium-rich foods?
>>
>> …los alimentos ricos en potasio?
>>
>> iv. Phosphorus-rich foods?
>>
>> …los alimentos ricos en fósforo?

77. Have you ever had a stroke?

¿Tuvo alguna vez un derrame cerebral [ataque cerebral/infarto cerebral/fallo cerebral/accidente cerebro vascular]? [¿Sufrió una apoplejía?]

> a. [If yes] When did you have a stroke?
>
> ¿Cuándo tuvo el derrame? [¿Cuándo sufrió la apoplejía?]

b. Did the stroke leave
lasting damage?
¿Le dejó daños permanentes
el derrame cerebral?

c. Show me where there is
a problem.
¿Muéstreme el problema?

78. Have you ever been told that diabetes has
damaged your eyes?

¿Le han dicho alguna vez que la diabetes le ha
afectado los ojos?

79. Do you need to put drops in your eyes?

¿Le hace falta echarse gotas en los ojos?

80. Do you wear glasses or contacts?

¿Usa anteojos [gafas, espejuelos] o lentes
de contacto?

81. Have you ever had surgery on your eyes?

¿Le han operado de los ojos alguna vez? [¿Le
han hecho cirugía en los ojos alguna vez?]

a. [If yes] Was it laser surgery or
conventional surgery?
¿Se trataba de cirugía con láser o
de cirugía tradicional?

82. When did you have surgery on your eyes?

¿Cuándo le operaron de los ojos?

83. Do you have any problems with your feet?

¿Tiene problemas en los pies?

84. Have you ever had a foot exam?

¿Se ha examinado de los pies alguna vez?

85. Do you have feeling in all parts of your feet?

¿Tiene sensación [sensibilidad] en todas las partes de los pies?

86. Have you ever had any surgery on your feet?

¿Le han operado alguna vez de los pies?

87. Have you had problems taking your medications as prescribed by your doctor?

¿Ha tenido problemas al tomar los medicamentos que le receta su médico?

88. Are you able to buy all the medications prescribed by your doctor?

¿Tiene los medios para comprarse todos los medicamentos que le receta su médico?

89. Do you know what all of your medications are for?

¿Sabe para qué sirven todos sus medicamentos?

Review of Systems (ROS)

90. Do you have any problems with your skin?

    ¿Tiene problemas de la piel?

91. Do you have any skin rashes or skin lesions? Would you show me?

    ¿Tiene sarpullidos o lesiones en la piel? ¿Me los puede enseñar?

92. Have you noticed a change in your vision?

    ¿Ha notado cambios en la vista?

    a. [If yes] When did this start?

    ¿Cuándo empezó?

93. Are your eyes blurry at times?

    ¿Se le ponen borrosos los ojos a veces?

94. Do your eyes tear often?

    ¿Le lloran a menudo los ojos?

95. Are your eyes dry?

    ¿Tiene los ojos resecos?

96. When was the last eye exam you had where they put drops in both eyes?

    ¿Cuándo se hizo el último examen de los ojos en que le pusieron gotas en los dos ojos?

97. Do you have any pain in your mouth?

    ¿Le duele la boca?

a. [If yes] How long have you had this pain?

¿Hace cuánto le duele?

98. Do you have any tooth pain?

¿Le duelen los dientes?

a. [If yes] How long have you had tooth pain?

¿Hace cuánto le duelen los dientes?

99. Do you have an infection in any of your teeth or mouth?

¿Tiene alguna infección en los dientes o en la boca?

100. Have you lost any of your teeth?

¿Le faltan dientes?

101. Do you have difficulty swallowing?

¿Se le hace difícil tragar?

a. [If yes] How long have you had difficulty swallowing?

¿Hace cuánto tiempo se le hace difícil tragar?

b. Do you have more difficulty swallowing hard foods or liquids?

¿Se le hace más difícil tragar alimentos duros o líquidos?

102. When was the last time you went to a dentist to have your teeth examined?

¿Cuándo fue la última vez que fue al dentista a examinarse los dientes?

103. Do you have a cough?
¿Tiene tos?

104. Are you coughing up phlegm?
¿Le sale flema al toser?

    a. [If yes] What is the color of the phlegm you are coughing up?
    ¿De qué color es la flema que le sale al toser?

105. Do you have a fever?
¿Tiene fiebre?

106. What has your temperature been?
¿En cuánto ha estado su temperatura?

107. Do you have a thermometer to take your temperature?
¿Tiene termómetro para tomarse la temperatura?

108. Are you having sweats or chills?
¿Le han dado sudores o escalofríos?

109. Do you have chest pain?
¿Tiene dolor de pecho?

    a. [If yes] How long have you had the pain?
    ¿Hace cuánto le duele?

b. Where exactly is the pain? Please point on your body.

¿Dónde le duele exactamente? Señálemelo con el dedo.

c. Does the chest pain move or go anywhere, or does it stay in one spot?

¿El dolor de pecho cambia de sitio o se queda en el mismo sitio?

d. What makes the pain appear?

¿Qué le da el dolor?

  i. Physical activity or exertion?

  ¿La actividad física o hacer esfuerzos?

  ii. Coughing?

  ¿Toser?

  iii. Heavy breathing?

  ¿Respirar fuerte?

e. What makes the pain go away? Aspirin, Tylenol, ibuprofen?

¿Qué le quita el dolor? ¿La aspirina, el Tylenol, el ibuprofeno?

110. Do you have shortness of breath?

¿Tiene problemas de falta de aliento (respiración)?

a. [If yes] How long have you had shortness of breath?

¿Hace cuánto tiempo tiene problemas de falta de aliento?

b. What are you doing when you get short of breath?

¿Qué hacía cuando tenía falta de aliento?

111. [For men] Do you have trouble getting an erection?

¿Tiene problemas para obtener la erección?

112. Do you feel you have difficulty digesting your food?

¿Cree tener dificultad para digerir alimentos?

113. Do you get heartburn?

¿Le da ardor de estómago [acidez estomacal]?

114. Do your ankles, fingers, or other parts of your body swell or become swollen?

¿Se le hinchan los tobillos, los dedos u otras partes del cuerpo?

a. [If yes] Show me on your body where you are swollen.

Muéstreme qué parte del cuerpo se le hincha?

b. Do you notice this after you sit for
   a long time?

   ¿Nota la hinchazón después de
   permanecer sentado (-a)
   mucho tiempo?

c. Does putting your feet up help?

   ¿Le sirve de alivio poner las
   piernas en alto?

115. Do you inspect, examine, or check your feet
every day?

¿Se inspecciona, examina o revisa los pies
todos los días?

116. Are there any red areas, blisters, or calluses on
your feet?

¿Tiene áreas rojas, ampollas o callos en
los pies?

117. Do you have any cuts or any infection on
your feet?

¿Tiene cortaduras o infecciones en los pies?

118. Do you put lotion on your feet every day?

¿Se pone loción en los pies todos los días?

119. Do you always wear shoes or slippers on
your feet?

¿Siempre lleva puestos zapatos o chanclas
[chancletas, chinelas, pantuflas, sandalias]?

120. Do you experience tingling or numbness of your feet?

¿Siente hormigueo [cosquilleo] o entumecimiento en los pies?

121. When was the last time a doctor examined your feet?

¿Cuándo fue la última vez que le examinó los pies un médico?

122. I would like to:

Quisiera…

   a. … check your height and weight.
   …ver que peso y estatura tiene.

   b. … check your waist size.
   …medirle la cintura.

   c. … check your blood glucose.
   …verificar su glucosa en la sangre.

   d. … see you check your blood glucose with your meter.
   …verle verificar su glucosa en la sangre con su medidor.

   e. … check your blood pressure
   …tomarle la presión.

   f. … check your pulse.
   …tomarle el pulso.

   g. … look into your eyes.
   …verle los ojos.

   h. … listen to your heart.
   …escucharle el corazón.

   i. … listen to your lungs.
   …escucharle los pulmones.

j. …examine your mouth.
   …examinarle la boca.

k. …examine your neck.
   …examinarle el cuello.

l. …examine your abdomen.
   …examinarle el abdomen.

m. …check your feet.
   …verle los pies.

123. Please take off your shoes and socks.

   Quítese los zapatos y los calcetines [las medias], por favor.

124. Please open your mouth wide.

   Abra bien la boca, por favor.

125. Please hold your breath.

   Aguante la respiración, por favor.

126. Please take deep breaths in and out.

   Aspire y exhale profundamente, por favor.

127. I would like to do a monofilament test by touching your foot with this wire. Please say "yes" whenever you feel the wire.

   Quisiera hacerle la prueba del monofilamento en la que le tocaré el pie con este alambre. Por favor diga "sí" cuando sienta el alambre.

128. Have you had a flu vaccine this year?

    ¿Se ha vacunado contra la gripe?

    a. [If no] May we give you a flu
       vaccine today?

       ¿Me permitiría vacunarle contra
       la gripe hoy?

129. Have you ever had a pneumonia vaccination?

    ¿Se ha vacunado contra la pulmonía?

    a. [If no] May we give you a
       pneumonia vaccination today?

       ¿Me permitiría vacunarle contra
       la pulmonía hoy?

130. Your next appointment will be…

    Su próxima cita será…

131. Do you use a pill box?

    ¿Utiliza una cajita de píldoras [caja para
    píldoras (pastillas)/ pastillero]?

132. You will be getting a new medication.

    Va a empezar a tomar un
    medicamento nuevo.

133. Please take your new medication this way…

    Por favor, tome el medicamento nuevo de
    esta manera…

134. You will be getting a blood test before your next appointment.

Se le hará una prueba de sangre antes de su próxima cita.

135. You will be getting an x-ray before your next appointment.

Se le sacarán radiografías [placas, rayos X] antes de su próxima cita.

136. Do you or your family have any questions?

¿Tienen alguna pregunta usted o su familia?

Special Situations: Prenatal Care and Preconception Counseling

Initial Questions and Concerns

137. Did you have diabetes before you were pregnant?

    ¿Tenía diabetes antes del embarazo?

    a. [If yes] Did you have type one diabetes or type two diabetes?

    ¿Tenía diabetes tipo uno o tipo dos?

138. How many weeks pregnant are you?

    ¿Cuántas semanas lleva de embarazo?

139. What is your due date?

    ¿Cuál es la fecha prevista de parto? [¿Para qué fecha se espera el bebé?]

140. What medications do you take?

    ¿Qué medicamentos toma?

    [Refer to List of Diabetes Medications for possible Spanish drug name variants]

141. Do you take prenatal vitamins?

    ¿Toma vitaminas prenatales (durante el embarazo)?

142. You need to take good care of your diabetes while pregnant to reduce the chances of:

Necesita cuidarse bien de la diabetes durante el embarazo para reducir la posibilidad de que…

   a. … your baby developing birth defects.

   …su bebé presente anomalías congénitas [defectos de nacimiento].

   b. … your baby having hypoglycemia after birth.

   …su bebé tenga hipoglucemia después del nacimiento.

   c. … your baby being too big at birth.

   …su bebé sea demasiado grande al nacer.

   d. … your baby developing jaundice.
   …su bebé contraiga ictericia.

   e. … your baby having problems breathing.

   …su bebé tenga problemas respiratorios.

   f. … you having a miscarriage.
   …usted tenga un aborto espontáneo [mal parto].

Glucose Monitoring

143. Do you have a meter to test your blood glucose?

    ¿Tiene un medidor de glucosa en la sangre?

    a. [If no] I would like to give you a meter to test and teach you how to use it.

       Le daré un medidor para que pruebe y para enseñarle el modo de usarlo.

144. You need to test your blood glucose before you eat (fasting), and one or two hours after you start eating your meal.

    Necesita verificar la glucosa en la sangre antes de comer (ayuno) y una o dos horas después de empezar sus comidas.

145. You will record your blood glucose values in this book.

    Apuntará los resultados en este registro.

146. I have circled the times to test your glucose.

    He trazado un círculo alrededor de las horas en que debe verificar la glucosa.

147. Bring your logbook to all of your medical appointments.

    Traiga el registro a todas sus citas médicas.

148. Your blood sugar should be less than ninety five milligrams per deciliter when you have not eaten and below one hundred twenty milligrams per deciliter one or two hours after eating.

Su azúcar en la sangre debe ser de menos de noventa y cinco miligramos por decilitro si no ha comido y estar por debajo de los ciento veinte miligramos por decilitro una o dos horas después de comer.

149. Tell your family you need to test your blood glucose four (five, six, seven) times per day.

Dígale a su familia que usted necesita verificar su glucosa en la sangre cuatro (cinco, seis, siete) veces al día.

150. Do you need to learn to take insulin?

    ¿Necesita aprender el modo de inyectarse la insulina?

    a. [If yes] You will be learning to take NPH insulin.

        Aprenderá a administrarse la insulina isofónica, NPH (letters pronounced in Spanish: ene, pé, ache).

    b. Here is the instruction book we will use.

        Éste es el manual de aprendizaje que utilizaremos.

151. You will be on Humalog/Novolog/Apidra insulin.

    Estará tomando insulina Humalog/Novolog/Apidra.

152. You will take your insulin before breakfast.

    Tomará la insulina antes del desayuno.

153. You will take your insulin at _____ PM/AM. [For 1 o'clock]

    Tomará la insulina a la una PM/AM.

[For other times]

Tomará la insulina a las dos (2) [tres (3), cuatro (4), cinco (5), seis (6), siete (7), ocho (8), nueve (9), diez (10), once (11), doce (12)] PM/AM.

154. You will take your insulin before lunch.

Tomará la insulina antes del almuerzo.

155. You will take your insulin before dinner.

Tomará la insulina antes de la cena.

156. Losing weight will help you have a healthier pregnancy.

Perder peso le ayudará a tener un embarazo saludable.

157. Your healthy weight is _____.

Su peso saludable es de _____.

158. Do you exercise?

¿Hace ejercicio?

    a. [If so] When?
      ¿Cuándo?

    b. How much?
      ¿Cuánto?

159. I would like you to start walking 30 minutes every day. If this is too much to begin with, start at 10 minutes per day and increase it every few days.

Quisiera que empiece a caminar trienta minutos al día. Si es demasiado para empezar, comience con diez minutos al día y aumente el tiempo a intervalos de unos cuantos días.

160. Your exercise should be low impact; walking is a good option.

El ejercicio que haga debe ser de poco impacto; caminar es una buena opción.

161. Do you follow any special food plan?

¿Sigue algún plan alimenticio especial?

162. Have you seen a dietitian?

¿Ha visto a un dietista?

a. [If no] You should see a dietitian and develop a healthy meal plan.

Debería ver a un dietista para desarrollar un plan de comidas saludable.

Spanish Diabetes Phrasebook

163. What birth control are you using?

¿Qué método usa para prevenir el embarazo?
[¿Qué tipo de anticonceptivos utiliza?]

164. Do you need to know the kinds of birth control available?

¿Necesita conocer los tipos de anticonceptivos que están disponibles?

165. You need to make sure your blood glucose levels are normal before you get pregnant again.

Es necesario que se asegure que los niveles de glucosa en la sangre sean normales antes de quedar embarazada otra vez.

166. Do you want any more children after this baby is born?

¿Quiere tener más niños después de que nazca éste?

List of Diabetes Medications

Oral medications

Metformin (Glucophage)
  metformina

Glipizide (Glucotrol)
  glipizida

Glyburide (Micronase/DiaBeta/Glynase/
PresTab)
  glibenclamida

Glimepiride (Amaryl)
  glimepirida

Pioglitazone (Actos)
  pioglitazona

Rosiglitazone (Avandia)
  rosiglitazona

Repaglinide (Prandin)
  repaglinida

Nateglinide (Starlix)
  nateglinida

Acarbose (Precose)
  acarbosa

Miglitol (Glyset)
   miglotol

Sitagliptin (Januvia)
   sitagliptina

Saxagliptin (Onglyza)
   saxagliptina

Injected medications—Insulin

Aspart (Novolog)
   asparta [aspártica, aspart]

Lispro (Humalog)
   lispro

Glulisine (Apidra)
   glulisina

Regular (Humulin R, Novolin R)
   regular

NPH (Humulin N, Novolin N)
   isofónica

Detemir (Levemir)
   detemir

Glargine (Lantus)
   glargina

Injected medications—Incretin Mimetics

Exenatide (Byetta)
    exenatida

Pramlintide (Symlin)
    pramlintida

Numbers

One	Uno
Two	Dos
Three	Tres
Four	Quatro
Five	Cinco
Six	Seis
Seven	Siete
Eight	Ocho
Nine	Nueve
Ten	Diez
Eleve	Once
Twelve	Doce
Thirteen	Trece
Fourteen	Catorce
Fifteen	Quince
Sixteen	Dieciséis
Seventeen	Diecisiete
Eighteen	Dieciocho
Nineteen	Diecinueve
Twenty	Veinta
Thirty	Treinta
Forty	Cuarenta
Fifty	Cincuenta
Sixty	Sesenta
Seventy	Setenta
Eighty	Ochenta
Ninety	Noventa
One hundred	Cien

List of Relevant Terms

A

Allergies
  Alergias

Ankle
  Tobillo

Arm
  Brazo

B

Black
  Negro (-a, -os, -as)

Bladder
  Vejiga

Blood
  Sangre

Blood glucose meter
  Medidor de glucosa en la sangre

Breast
  Pecho [seno (of a woman)]

Brown
    Marrón [castaño (-a, -os, -as), of hair—
    moreno (-a, -os, -as), of skin]

C

Cancer
    Cáncer

Calf
    Pantorrilla

Cheek
    Mejilla

Chest
    Pecho

Colors
    Colores

> Black
>   Negro (-a, -os, -as)
>
> White
>   Blanco (-a, -os, -as)
>
> Gray
>   Gris
>
> Brown
>   Marrón [castaño (-a, -os, -as) café, of
>   hair—moreno (-a, -os, -as), of skin]

Red
    Rojo (-a, -os, -as)

Blue
    Azul (-es)

Green
    Verde (-es)

Orange
    Anaranjado (-a, -os, -as)

Yellow
    Amarillo (-a, -os, -as)

Violet
    Violeta (-as)

Purple
    Púrpura (-as)

Cornea
Córnea

D

Diabetes
    Diabetes

Dietary supplements
    Suplementos [complementos] dietéticos

Dietitian
    Dietista

Doctor
   Médico [doctor].

Dosage
   Dosis

Drugs
   Medicamentos (medicine); drogas (narcotic)

E

Ear
   Oreja

Elbow
   Codo

Erectile dysfunction
   Disfunción erectil

Esophagus
   Esófago

Exercise physiologist
   Fisiólogo (-a) de ejercicios

Eye
   Ojo

Eye lid
   Párpado

F

Finger
  Dedo

Finger nail
  Uña del dedo

Flu
  Gripe

Food
  Alimento

Foot
  Pie

G

Gall bladder
  Vesícula biliar

Gestational
  Gestacional [gravídico, del embarazo]

Glucose
  Glucosa [azúcar]

Green
  Verde (-es)

Hair
Pelo [Cabello]

Hand
Mano

Head
Cabeza

Head cold
Resfriado

Heart
Corazón

Heart attack
Ataque al corazón [cardíaco]/
infarto cardíaco /fallo cardíaco

Help
Ayuda

Herbs
Hierbas

Infection
Infección

Injection
Inyección

Spanish Diabetes Phrasebook

Insulin
    Insulina

Intestine
    Intestino

Intravenous
    Intravenoso (-a, -os, -as)

K

Kidney
    Riñón

Knee
    Rodilla

L

Leg
    Pierna

Liver
    Hígado

Lungs
    Pulmones

M

Medical record
    Historial médico
    [registro/record médico]

Medicine
    Medicamento [medicina]

Mouth
    Boca

N

Nose
    Nariz

Nurse
    Enfermero (-a)

Nurse practitioner
    Enfermera (-o) de práctica avanzada [enfermera
    (-o) universitaria]

Nutritionist
    Nutricionista [especialista en nutrición,
    nutrióloga (-o)]

P

Pancreas
    Páncreas

Penis
    Pene

Phlegm
    Flema

Physician assistant
    Asociado [Auxiliar, Asistente] médico

Pill
    Píldora [Pastilla]

Pulse
    Pulso

R

Red
    Rojo (-a, -os, -as)

Retina
    Retina

S

Saline solution
    Solución salina

Shin
    Espinilla

Skin
    Piel

Stomach
Estómago [Barriga]

Stroke
Derrame cerebral [apoplejía]

Surgery
Cirugía

Swallow
Tragar

T

Teeth
Dientes

Tears
Lagrimas

Throat
Garganta

Thumb
Pulgar

Toe
Dedo del pie

Toe nail
Uña del dedo del pie

Tooth
Diente

Type
    Tipo

U

Urine
    Orina

Urethra
    Uretra

V

Vagina
    Vagina

Vision
    Vista

Vitamins
    Vitaminas

W

Water
    Agua

White
    Blanco (-a, -os, -as)

Wrist
    Muñeca

X

X-ray
Radiografía [placa, rayos X]

Y

Yeast Infection:
infección fúngica [infección por hongos o
micosis, infección vaginal, Candidiasis o
Cándida vulvovaginitis, hongos deuteromicetes
patógenos, hongo del género Cándida]

Yellow
Amarillo (-a, -os, -as)